**Paste Your Inspirational Photo**
**In frame below**
**For instructions see Tool Box #2**

Insert Photo here

# MY DOIN' IT WORKBOOK

### By Kit DeCanti

## Published By KitDee productions

>^..^<

## Copyright Carolyn DeCanti 2011

For information contact KitDee Productions at:

marketing@kitdeeproductions.com

For reviews and comments from readers and more information about author and other books

written by Kit DeCanti go to:

http:www.kitdeeproductions.com

Most books by Kit DeCanti are available at special quantity

discounts for bulk purchases for sales promotions, premiums or

fund raising. Special books or book excerpts can also be created

to fit specific needs.

ISBN-13: 978-1463559168 and

ISBN-10: 146355916x

First printing: November 2011 Printed in the U.S.A.

Dedicated to my support team,
Sue Little, Kathleen Rogers, Dar
Brown, Jessyca Rogers, Janice
Heinzelman, Ruth Hyde, Jeanie
Hall, & Kathy Hess…
And to all the woman who have
been carrying around heavy
baggage and want to know how
to shed it- I'm also dedicating
this book to YOU!

Give yourself the gift of your
heart's desire-
Only YOU can make you
thin.
Remember
NOTHING TASTES AS
GOOD AS HAPPY,
HEALTHY, ENERGETIC,
THIN & STRONG FEELS!

# MY SUPPORT TEAM

(Read Tool Box #13 before choosing your Support Team)

| NAME | PHONE # | EMAIL ADDRESS |
|------|---------|---------------|
| Kit DeCanti | (707) 350-1967 | kit@kitdeeproductions.com |
|  |  |  |
|  |  |  |
|  |  |  |
|  |  |  |
|  |  |  |
|  |  |  |
|  |  |  |
|  |  |  |
|  |  |  |
|  |  |  |
|  |  |  |
|  |  |  |
|  |  |  |
|  |  |  |
|  |  |  |
|  |  |  |
|  |  |  |
|  |  |  |
|  |  |  |
|  |  |  |
|  |  |  |
|  |  |  |
|  |  |  |

# Table Of Contents

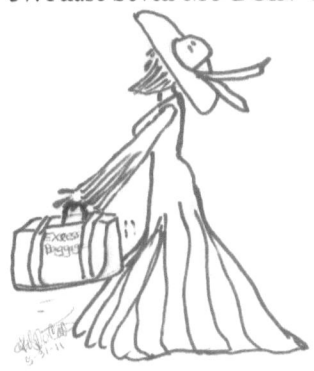

## Disclaimer

Before starting this or any weight loss plan talk to your medical doctor to make sure that you are healthy enough to go on a plan without the supervision of a doctor.

The author and publisher of this book in no way are representing themselves as being in the medical field or experts on the subject of nutrition or weight loss. The author is only sharing information that she has gathered over several years of yo-yo dieting. After years of failing to shed the excess baggage she was carrying on her small frame, and which was contributing to her bad health; she devised and implemented a plan that worked for her. She is sharing that plan with you.

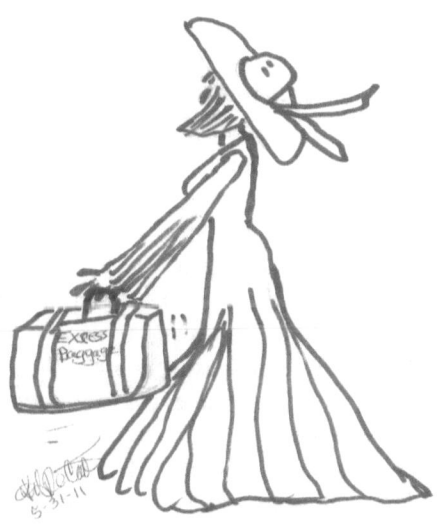

# Introduction

**MY DOIN' PLAN** is just that- a plan that YOU can personalize into what works for you to finally DO IT. To finally get off the yo-yo dieting, extreme regimes, fads, and everything else that you've tried and that failed you. They failed you because it was someone else's' plan. Someone else's regime. But here is a fact that I came to understand to be true: We all want to be fit, thin and healthy. It is our heart's desire. But here is the point- Only YOU can give yourself the gift of your heart's desire Only YOU can make you thin. As true as that statement is it is also true that you need a tool belt full of tools at your disposal in order to fine tune yourself mentally, emotionally and physically in order to build that precious gift to yourself. I have spent years researching and gathering information until finally I got it. I got it! I got the point that I needed to stop trying to copy someone else's success story. I needed to write my own. And along the way I gathered enough tools to do just that! In order to use those tools I needed a good personalized tool box to keep them in. This book is just *that*. A tool box with some excellent tools, but with space compile your own tools as you gather them. I've enclosed some that I found helpful. You can use them or not as fits your personal situation and life.

Does the DOIN' IT PLAN really work? Well, see for your self. On the next page are before and after photos of me- Kit DeCanti. The before was taken two weeks before starting the DOIN' IT plan and the after was taken less than 6 months later. Forty Plus pounds lighter! …. This workbook got me there! And is helping me shed even more excess baggage & pounds.

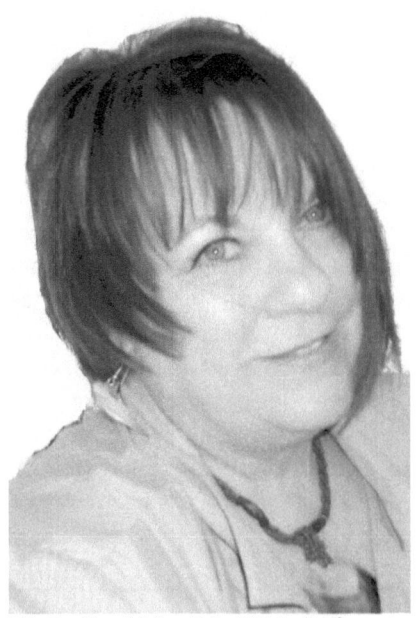

Kit DeCanti May 7th 2011 -Before starting Doin' It

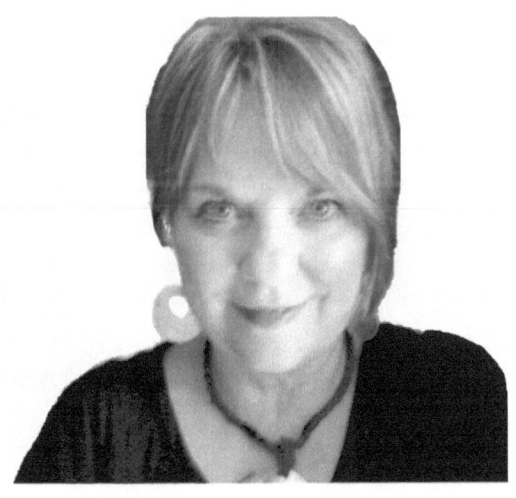

Kit DeCanti After Doin' It for 5 Months~ Oct /15th 20/11
(*for a complete photo record of her journey see back page)

# TOOL BOX

## #1 Reasons

The first tool you need in your tool box is Reasons. We all have different reasons for picking up this book. Sure we all want to be healthy, fit and thin. That's our *goal*. But we need motivation to get us on- and keep us on- the road to that goal. List the reasons you want and NEED to stay on that road below: (Such as physical & emotional health, heart healthier, live longer, more energy, breathing easier, certain- and be specific- activities easier, look better, more self confidence, wear styles you love... what ever will motivate and inspire YOU to get started and stay on the road to Thin & Healthy.)

_____

_____

_____

_____

_____

_____

_____

_____

_____

_____

_____

_____

_____

_____

_____

_____

_____

_____

## #2 Motivations & Inspirations

Another tool to help get you motivated to start your plan, and to keep you going, you also need to be 'Inspired' and to be 'Motivated'; and words are a tool that can do that for you.

There are plenty of inspirational sayings and slogans to adapt to your personal situation.

I've inserted my two favorites at the beginning of this book. Another phrase I love is "Face It, Trace It, Erase It, Replace It" (which is Tool #10). List your favorites here (and add more as you work your plan:

_____

_____

_____

_____

_____

_____

_____

_____

_____

_____

_____

_____

_____

_____

_____

_____

_____

_____

_____

_____

_____

_____

_____

## #3 Inspiration Photo

You are no doubt familiar with the term "A picture is worth a thousand words." Well in the case of weight loss a picture is worth a dozen pounds (or more). I found a photo to inspire me and it helped me shed dozens of pounds. What would inspire you? Perhaps a photo of yourself before giving birth; one before years of comforting yourself with food- padding yourself from fearful situations... real or imagined. Or it could be the body you want with your face digitally inserted. That is what I did. Sure I had plenty of thin photos of myself from years ago- but I found that they only made sadness and guilt well up inside me and before I knew it I was binging. But a current photo of my face on the body I want to give myself was just what I needed. What ever *feels right* for you *will work for you.* Tape your inspirational photo on the first page of this book. Of course there are more tools to put in your tool box. And girl do I have them for you! Keep reading.

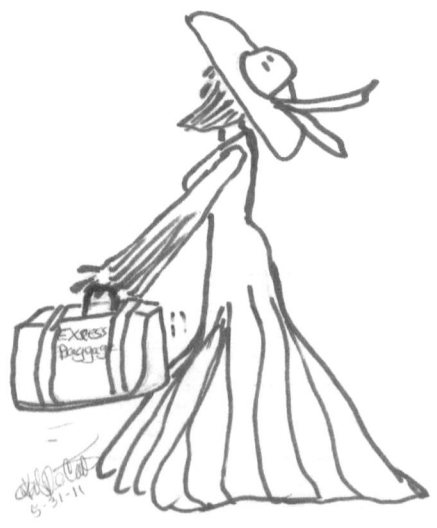

## #4 Words

Something that has a huge impact on us humans are 'Words'… they can be an important and helpful tool. They can also be a weapon to stumble us off the road to Healthy, Fit, Thin, and Strong. We need to change the way we talk. To others and especially to our ourselves. To YOU. You need to talk kinder to yourself and about yourself. I know I know- you are going to read in Phase One the word 'fat' and while it's true that we must get real with ourselves and where our body is now- we need not call our selves hurtful things. Instead **use words to comfort yourself.** There are also terms that may bring up hurtful, fearful or uncomfortable emotions or thoughts. Words like 'losing'. Or 'lost'. I mean it's a no-brainer- who wants to 'lose' anything? Let alone a part of yourself. Most people who are carrying the heavy load of extra pounds are having a difficult time trying to find them selves in all the *excess baggage* that they carry. Sometimes it is because of the extra weight but most of the time the baggage is causing the excess weight. I fit in that category. I have found it very helpful to replace the word 'losing' and 'lost' with 'shedding' and 'shed'. I have shed 50+ pounds without losing myself with them. I actually was able to find myself as I shed those heavy pounds. With the help of a few more tools I also shed tons of emotional baggage. More on that later.

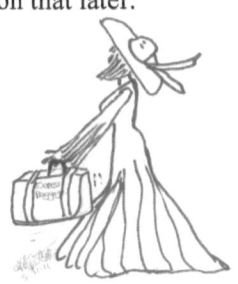

## #5 Doing What Comes Naturally- or Should!

To shed the pounds you want to, you need to Breath, Start Moving, and Drinking Water. Sounds simple, doesn't it? Yes these normal activities that we were designed to do but are also activities that people carrying excess weight and baggage have a tendency to neglect giving themselves. Let's take some time to think about them one at a time.

## #6 Start Breathing

Right now! Step back and take a deep breath. May not be as easy as it sounds. You probably have been holding your breath or making a habit of only taking shallow breaths without even realizing it. So you need to learn how to breath properly. How to breath the way our bodies were designed to breath. To fill our lungs with life giving oxygen that will be absorbed by the lungs and picked up by our blood vessels to replenishing our cells. First you need to blow out all the excess stale air in your lungs. Now hold it for a few moments. Okay, now your lungs are ready to accept the gift you are about to give them. You now can breath deeply into the far corners that have not been enriched with pure clean oxygen for probably some time. Feels good doesn't it? Do it again. Feel the oxygen enter your blood stream energizing yet relaxing you. Do this often. As often as you remember. And especially every time you start to feel uptight or stressed. Remember this tool. Keep it handy! Now lets move on to the next tool...

## #7 Moving

Don't just sit there MOVE! Every time you move you increase the number of fat (there's that word again) cells that you eliminate from your wonderful body. You move closer to 'Thinsville'. Standing burns more than sitting. And moving burns more that just standing. And the more you move the better you will feel inside and out! Move for the joy of moving! Walk, jog, dance, skate, row, ski, swim, bike, tennis, volley ball, hop scotch! Anything as long as it makes you smile. Better yet laugh- laughing is a great way to lift your spirits while lifting fat off your abs. Moving will also help you with Tool #6- Breathing. It will also make you thirsty. Which brings us to the next Tool.

**#8 Drink Water**
Are you one of the people that think that if you drink coffee, sodas, milk, juice etc you don't need to drink water? Think again! We are designed to drink water! We need it!! It is recommended by most experts that you stop (or at least drastically reduce) your coffee, tea & soda intake. In fact for every ounce of these substances you drink, you need to add that much (or more) of water to flush it out of your bodies. Our bodies are mostly water, and were designed to replenish water regularly. That means daily. Many experts say that drinking 1/3 – 1/2 of our body weight in ounces of water can aid in shedding excess weight. I have found this to be true. Amazingly true. And In fact what is amazing is that for people who are retaining water (like myself) it takes water to flush it out of the system. And shedding that excess water shows up as lower numbers on the bathroom scales, and measuring tape.
Oh yes- those are other important tool.

## #9 SCALES & Measuring Tape.

Make friends with the dreaded bathroom scales.

To know where you are going you need to know where you are. So the scales and measuring tape needs to be part of your tool box.

I used to hate my scales. I avoided it. I hid it. I covered it with a magazine basket. But when I made friends with it, I found it was my favorite tool. Make your scales your friend. It's a friend that won't lie to you to spare your feelings. It will tell you the truth to keep you on your program. It won't call you names, it just states the facts in a non accusing, non judgmental and private manner. It respects your feelings. It will be honest and open with you and will be the first one to give you the good news. You are shedding weight. You will find yourself in a hurry to greet your new friend first thing each morning. Well- the

$2^{nd}$ thing. First you need to, ah-hem, use the toilette (sounds more polite in French). You will also need to measure yourself once a week. This will be an invaluable tool when you've reached a plateau and need reassurance that you are making progress. You will find a couple places to record your measurements in this book (later). Copy your measurements into your journal (Tool #13 and discussed more in Phase Two). Then continue to measure yourself weekly or at least monthly and record the results in your journal.

## #10 Goals and Rewards

These are two extremely valuable tools but I won't talk too much about it here because it is Phase Five, and it is discussed in detail then. I will only say that to get where we want to go we need a map. A starting place and a destination- or goal. And we also need a gage to measure our success. And as humans need positive reinforcement to succeed and continue to succeed. And no one can give YOU exactly what YOU want but YOU. Not just one big reward at the end of your journey to thinness, but setting smaller easier to reach goals has yielded great success in many controlled research programs. And although we want to keep the ultimate 'prize' in mind we should focus more on the short term, reachable goals- one at a time. Really celebrate each goal as you reach them. You are in control of how many points for each goal (or if you use the point system or not) and what the reward will be (Rewards are a MUST!). Make the rewards something YOU really want and that will make YOU happy. After all YOU earned it!

## #11 Solutions for Triggers

Ever have a frustrating day at work, a fight with your spouse or close friend, bad day with the kids- then end up cozying up with a nice cold pint of chocolate-chip ice cream? Of course. We've *all* been going strong on a program, when BAM! We hit a wall! That wall is called 'Triggers'. It can come in many forms. And no matter what direction we go, we will hit another wall. More triggers. *It's inevitable.* It's important to understand and accept that fact. But we need not succumb or be stumbled from our goal of becoming healthy, fit and trim. We just need to recognize the triggers and see how we have handled them in the past and choose a new way of handling them and to have it at our fingertips- in our 'Tool Box'. In other words we need to be prepared. I've prepared a list of triggers and solutions. It will become one of your greatest tools. It will help you think each situation out as well as help you as new walls pop up. At the end of my list, there is space to add others you think of or as they appear:

**TRIGGER:** Frustrated because there is something that I WANT or want to do and I feel stagnated because something/someone prevents it.

**FEELING:** Anxious, anger, nervous, jittery, can't think, false hunger, cravings

**THOUGHTS:** Thoughts of food, blame, self derogating words

**OLD ACTION:** Blame self, blame others, out burst, yell, argue, then blame self for fighting with others, derogatory words, 'munch' or binge

**OLD REACTION:** Guilt shame, disgust, self hate, blame, exhaustion, depression binging

**SOLUTION:** Breath, drink lemon water, journal or talk about it. Decide if it's really that important to do right now. If not set a future date for it, or forget about it. Ask yourself if it's worth throwing self away? What do you want the outcome to be? If it is really important NOW then announce the problem and anxious feelings because of need to do it and state that you are putting everything else on hold and DO IT.

**NEW REACTION:** Happy, relaxed, self satisfied, self pride,

**REWARD: 10 POINTS**

**TRIGGER:** Stressful day trying to get stuff done and no energy or just can't think

**FEELING:** Anxious, confused, darkness closing in, nervousness, false hunger, craving guilt

**THOUGHTS:** Thoughts of food, blame others, self blame, "I should...." hateful words to self or others

**OLD ACTION:** Binge, reach for junk food

**OLD REACTION:** Guilt shame, disgust, self hate, blame, exhaustion, more binging

**SOLUTION:** Breath, drink large glass of lemon water, make a list, cross off unimportant tasks, break job into doable sessions set timer for 30 min START and stop when time up, give self permission to keep going if you feel up to it- if not permission to take a non food break. If hunger is real reach for healthy snack or meal. Journal or talk about it.

**NEW REACTION:** Happy, relaxed, self satisfied, self pride

**REWARD: 10 POINTS**

**TRIGGER:** Been on program and shedding weight- everything is fine when SUDDEN cravings, old tapes and feelings from past or other strong emotions to come up.

**FEELING:** Overwhelming sadness and/or anxiousness, nervousness, food cravings, specific junk food craving, anger, tears, depression, guilt, shame

**THOUGHTS**: Blame self or others, hurtful words about self or others, thoughts of comfort foods

**Old REACTION:** Binge, munch, reach for junk food or seconds at next meal, angry yelling, crying,

**SOLUTION:** Breath, drink large glass of lemon water, journal or talk about it, let the tears come. Remember that you've lived through it and remembering it won't be the same as it happening again. Only way past it is through it. Hit a pillow. Write a letter to perpetrator, draw a picture and spit on it. Tear it to pieces and flush it. Yell, stomp, run- what ever it takes to get through and past the feelings and thoughts. Then say good by to it. It's over. Past. Done. You never have to live through it again.(If you are in an unsafe situation- get out of it now. There are agencies to help.)

**NEW REACTION:** Relief, happy, self pride satisfactions, confident accomplished, feel good, content, relaxed, comforted, self love

**REWARD: 10 POINTS**

**TRIGGERING EVENT:** Skipped previous meal
**FEELINGS:** Excessive hunger, shaky, light headed
**THOUGHTS:** Thoughts: I'm ravenous! Since I didn't eat breakfast, I can pig out at lunch. I skipped lunch so I take extra desert.
**OLD ACTIONS:** Eating fast and keep eating even when satisfied to make up for the meal you skipped
**OLD REACTIONS:** Guilt shame, disgust, self hate, blame, exhaustion, more binging
**SOLUTION:** Grab a piece of fruit as a snack or a handful of nuts to take the edge off. Wait 15 or 20 minutes, then eat from your program, taking care to eat slow. Resolve to eat regularly as per your program.
**NEW REACTION:** Feel good about self, happy, self satisfactions, accomplished, content, relaxed, comforted, satisfied
**REWARD: 10 POINTS**

**TRIGGERING EVENT:** Social gathering where you don't know anyone
**FEELINGS:** Self conscious, shy, nervous, anxious, uneasy, heart palpitations, sweaty, queasy stomach, bored,
**THOUGHTS :** "Why isn't anyone talking to me? I might as well occupy myself here by the snack table. Ahh comfort food, maybe some chips will settle my stomach."
**OLD ACTIONS:** Eating too much, Eating when not hungry, comforting self with food
**OLD REACTIONS:** Guilt, shame, disgust, self hate, blame, exhaustion, more binging
**SOLUTION:** Step away from the snack table, look

around for someone who is standing by herself and introduce yourself. Or ask the host to introduce you to a few people. Ask the hostess if you can help out, prepare self with mental list of conversation starters

**NEW REACTION:** Feel good about self, happy, self satisfactions, accomplished, content, relaxed, comforted, satisfied, self confident, happy to have made new friends

**REWARD: 10 POINTS**

**TRIGGERING EVENT:** A party or get together. (Can you say red velvet cupcakes?)

**FEELINGS:** Excited, happy, nervous, anxious, giddy

**THOUGHTS:** Thoughts: I've worked hard all day. I deserve a treat. I've been 'good' I can 'enjoy myself' for a change and restart tomorrow. I can't resist this. I can't pass up this opportunity. Can't pass up opportunity to try (Whatever temptation pops up)

**OLD ACTIONS:** Eat more than you need. Eat things not good for you. Eat too much. Scarfing down a cupcake (or two!) though you've just had lunch and are not hungry.

**OLD REACTIONS:** Guilt, shame, disgust, self hate, blame, exhaustion, more binging

**SOLUTION:** Realize that food is not disappearing off the planet. This is not your last meal. You will have plenty of other opportunities to eat it. Nothing tastes as good as healthy, fit, and thin feels. Ask yourself if you are prepared to trade your self esteem for it. Split a cupcake with a colleague. Enjoy it. Then join in an activity or seek out your favorite person there and distract yourself with good conversation until the party is over.

**NEW REACTION:** Feel good about self, happy,

self satisfactions, accomplished, content, relaxed, comforted, satisfied, elevated self esteem
**REWARD: 10 POINTS**

**TRIGGERING EVENT:** Everyone else around the table is having seconds. When you refuse, your mother/hostess asks, "What—you don't like it?!" or "Come on it won't hurt just this time. I made it especially for you! I want your opinion."
**FEELINGS:** Anger, uncomfortable, guilt, controlled, don't want to hurt feelings, in a corner, desire to fit in, feel used or controlled
**THOUGHTS:** I can't believe this is happening again! I guess it's better to give in than cause a scene. It was good. I can 'start again tomorrow' 'She/He's trying to control me again.'
**OLD ACTIONS:** Resentfully agree to another helping, followed by a double helping of regret.
**OLD REACTIONS:** Guilt shame, disgust, self hate, blame, exhaustion, more binging
**SOLUTION:** Tell your mom/hostess you loved it, let her know you're really full- then change the subject with a smile.
**NEW REACTION:** Happy, in control, satisfied, self confident, strong, Feel good about self, accomplished, content, relaxed, comforted, elevated self esteem and independance
**REWARD: 10 POINTS**

**TRIGGERING EVENT:** Ongoing problem at work/home/social circle
**FEELINGS:** Heart pounding, anger, feelings hurt, urge to run
**THOUGHTS:** I feel out of control. I feel inadequate, My feelings are hurt, he/she has no right

to say that or to treat me that way. I feel isolated left out, unloved.

**OLD ACTIONS:** You go out with spouse or friend to vent- and eat and/or drink way too much.

**OLD REACTIONS:** Guilt shame, disgust, self hate, blame, exhaustion, more binging

**SOLUTION:** Make a point of leaving situation on the early side for a few days running, take a walk or head to the gym, curl up on the couch and get engrossed in a novel or your favorite TV show or movie. Join spouse or a good friend for light dinner and one drink.

**NEW REACTION:** Feel good about self, happy, self satisfactions, accomplished, content, relaxed, comforted, satisfied

**REWARD: 10 POINTS**

**TRIGGERING EVENT:** You had a bad date/social event. Very bad!

**FEELINGS:** Sad, lonely, unloved, disgusted, angry

**THOUGHTS:** I'll never find anyone to love! Or good friend who likes me, Why am I always treated like that? I must be worthless. Who could love me?

**OLD ACTIONS:** Can you say chocolate?

**OLD REACTIONS:** Guilt shame, disgust, self hate, blame, depression, binging, exhaustion, more binging

**SOLUTION:** Call your most soothing friend to vent, then do something creative—write, knit, draw or whatever floats your boat. Remind yourself that you wouldn't have time to nurture your strengths if you were constantly catering to someone who didn't get you.

**NEW REACTION:** Feel good about self, happy,

self satisfactions, accomplished, content, relaxed, comforted, satisfied

**REWARD: 10 POINTS**

**TRIGGER:** Boss/spouse/someone else drops a last-minute project on your already overloaded plate.

**FEELINGS:** Emotions: Tense muscles, pounding heart, resentment, blame, anger, stress

**THOUGHTS:** I'm totally overwhelmed. I'll never get all this done. That lazy so & so never pulls their own weight! I need something to help me calm down/get through/give me strength

**OLD ACTIONS:** You stay late in the office/stay up late to finish and skip dinner, then make up for it by eating half the contents of your refrigerator later. Blame, outburst, binge

**OLD REACTIONS:** Guilt shame, disgust, self hate, blame, exhaustion, more binging

**SOLUTION:** Bring some work home so you can leave at a reasonable hour. Break task into smaller doable jobs. Ask for help. Before you have dinner (plan on something you really love, that feels luxurious but that's reasonable calorie wise and on your program—say, a fresh salad topped with grilled or broiled shrimp), then go for a walk, or turn up the music and dance around the living room to de-stress. Don't you feel better?

**NEW REACTION:** Relief, feel good about self, happy, self satisfied and accomplished, elevated self esteem, content, relaxed, comforted, satisfied

**REWARD: 10 POINTS**

**Now your turn:**
TRIGGER:_____
OLD REACTION:  _____

FEELING: _____

THOUGHTS: _____

SOLUTION:_____

NEW REACTION: _____

NEW FEELING: _____

REWARD POINTS:_____


TRIGGER:_____

OLD REACTION: _____

FEELING: _____

THOUGHTS: _____

SOLUTION:_____

NEW REACTION: _____

NEW FEELING: _____

REWARD POINTS:_____


TRIGGER:_____

OLD REACTION: _____

FEELING: _____

THOUGHTS: _____

SOLUTION:_____

NEW REACTION: _____

NEW FEELING: _____

REWARD POINTS:_____

TRIGGER:_____

OLD REACTION: _____

FEELING: _____

THOUGHTS: _____

SOLUTION:_____

NEW REACTION: _____

NEW FEELING: _____

REWARD POINTS:_____

TRIGGER:_____
OLD REACTION: _____
FEELING: _____
THOUGHTS: _____
SOLUTION:_____
NEW REACTION: _____
NEW FEELING: _____
REWARD POINTS:_____
**Note: These reward points are to be used only on things that will make YOU happy!! Because you're worth it!**

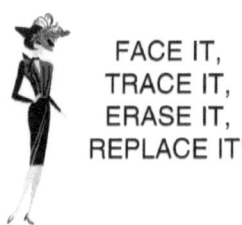

FACE IT,
TRACE IT,
ERASE IT,
REPLACE IT!

## #12 Face, Trace, Erases & Replace Emotions

All that talk about 'Feelings' brings us to another invaluable tool, that we need to understand. We need to know what makes you tick. What causes certain things to be triggers for you in the first place. Because you have many feelings on many levels that will make unconscious choices unless you recognize them. You need to be aware of that!

To recognize feelings you must make a conscience effort to feel them. In Phase 7 there is space to jot down those feelings. You may find it useful to copy the notes from this book into your journal (Phase 2)- and write about it in detail. You will realize some feelings that have been 'installed' at different times in your life that may be inappropriate now. However until you deal with them they will continue to control your thoughts, actions and decisions and choices.

Something that you may not know.... When ever you feel something VERY STRONG, that is have a strong reaction to an event, a comment, an action- it has more to do with the past than the present. Something from your past is triggering these strong emotions.

Points To Remember :

- **DON'T REACT....ACT**
    **Before making choices in life ask yourself:**
- **What will this choice produce?**

                        **and**

- **Am I willing and ready to accept the consequences (with out thinking I can control or change them)?**

**Once you take a breath and realize that there are other solutions to stress besides rampant binging, and that the choice is yours- you've got a good start on winning the battle of the bulge.**

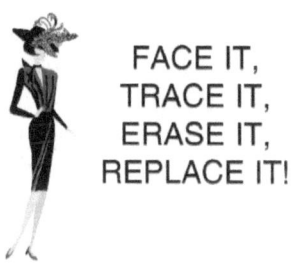

FACE IT,
TRACE IT,
ERASE IT,
REPLACE IT!

### #13 Journaling

Although Phase Two is Journaling, I've added it to your tool box to emphasize this invaluable tool. There is no way a person could be able to get to the root of and deal with an eating disorder without journaling, in my opinion (and other's). It is a *MUST*! We will discuss this more in Phase Two.

### #14 Food Facts

In Phase Four you pick YOUR plan. But I thought it

would be helpful to add some food facts to your tool box. I recommend that you stay clear of liquid cleanses. You won't get lasting results in your body. However, a cleanse is definitely needed. But I suggest eating your way clean! There are many veggies that will add a nutrient, and energy boost while will ridding your body of toxins; plus you won't be hungry and weak! Choose veggies that are high in alkaline. You will want to learn as much as you can about alkalizing yourself. It is the best thing you can do for your heath. Foods that are high in alkaline are not surprisingly foods that are famous for 'melting' fat from your body. A few of these are cucumbers, broccoli, spinach, lemons, almonds (raw preferably) sun flower seeds, and my fave- zucchini. Nothing blah about any of those. And the more of those you eat uncooked the more alkaline your body will become. A bonus benefit is your energy level will go through the roof! My favorite breakfast is Tomatoes, Cucumbers & Avocado Slices. Yes avocado- it is full of 'good healthy' fats that will help your skin keep it's elasticity while you shed unhealthy fat.

A great snack is Almonds & Cucumbers…. Soak the almonds over night in water, and discard the liquid. Peal & chop the cukes into squares and put in air tight container to carry with you, and munch to your heart's delight. And yes, your heart *will* be delighted!

An interesting study conducted among college students revealed that although all the students continued to eat as usual those who ADDED almonds to their daily diet shed weight. Not surprising since adding alkaline to your daily diet will help balance out the acid and so your body doesn't need the extra fat to protect you from all that acid you pour into yourself with the common American diet. (research it).

So here's the nitty gritty on detoxing- First off why is it important? Because the American way of eating fills our bodies with unhealthy processed foods, food additives, substitutes and poisons- yes poisons! The body tries to protect your arteries from these poisonous high acid poisons and VOILA cholesterol is born! Which also is very bad for your health! And what gets through your blood stream ends up on your hips, thighs, belly etc as 'cellulite'. These are fat cells that your body can't use because they are made up of toxins. How to get rid of it? You guessed it- Cleanse! First off skip added sugars. All sugar or sugar substitutes except ones made from the plant stevia. And avoid anything with high- fructose corn syrup like the plague!!! Next skip all the bad fats that are high in saturated fat. And if you don't love tofu yet- at least develop a friendly relationship! It's the best source of protein!! But white fish and a little chicken are good too. Oh and lay off the booze!! Toxic! (at least until you reach your goal!- and then drink sparingly) Don't forget fiber. As you can see you can comfortably and successfully 'eat your way to thin!' Oh Besides 'what' you eat you need to focus on 'how' you eat. To shed the pounds you need to also shed some bad habits- like gulping your food and eating on the run, or worse in front of the Boob Tube! Set a nice table, sit down and eat slowly. Take a bite, put down your fork. Chew slowly enjoying every taste and texture, swallow. Take a sip of Lemon water. (VERY alkaline- in fact, since it has no sugars, I rarely drink water with out lemon juice in it) Converse if you are eating with friends or family. Repeat.

Another interesting food fact is that it is better to eat six *small* meals than three large meals. I'm sure you know lots more food facts or can find them easily enough, so I won't spend any more time on that subject. This book is designed to help you stick to what ever plan YOU chose for yourself.

## #15 Support Team

We all need someone to lean on or a shoulder to cry on now and again. No matter how much we tend to try to keep our 'dieting' (sorry for using that dreaded word) secret, we all need a friend or two to be our confidant. We need a support team to cheer us on when we shed excess baggage, pounds and inches; and to comfort us when the emotional stuff comes up. And especially to encourage us to keep on 'Doin' It'! I put the form for your support team at the front of this book for easy access. These buddies can be chosen from your family, friends, workmates or the world wide web. Cyberspace is literally crawling with online support groups. Where ever you choose to pick your support group- be careful to choose wisely and safely.

Not everyone is going to be supportive. Another fact of life, some times people are saboteurs ...And with Friends like those .... well you know.

There will be some who won't want to lose their 'eating buddy' much like a drinker or smoker won't encourage their buddies to leave their circle. There will also be some who no matter how many pounds you shed will always want to make you the butt of their unkind jokes. And we can't overlook the well doers who will chime in unison "A little won't hurt you. You can start again tomorrow. or how about this familiar sabotage, " "Come on- I made this especially for you it's my specialty." As sad and discouraging as it is, we all have these people in our lives. So it is necessary to make a statement of your intentions. No

24

excuses. Your success depends on it. I've included the following form to insure that you do.

## #16 NOTIFICATION:
Put an 'X' in the appropriate box below:
I have notified those I live with and see each day of my intentions to eat a certain way, and asked them not to offer me anything off my plan
Y __N__ (this will help you identify saboteurs that you will need to deal with or avoid)

**Okay, you've loaded your tool box with enough ammunition to stave off any attack. You are now ready to officially start YOUR Doin' Plan.**

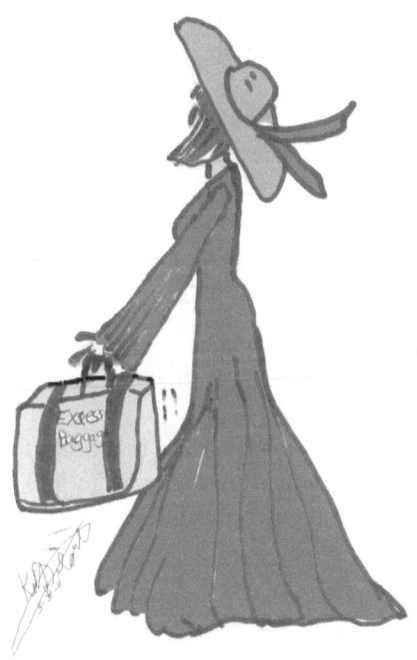

# DOIN' PLAN

## PHASE ONE
### Let's Get Honest

Record today's date, your weight and measurements here: Put today's date even though you haven't chosen or began your Doin' It plan yet. Well actually you have. The first part of this workbook was designed to help you get into the right frame of mind. And that is imperative to start 'Doin' It'.

And now for honesty. Getting honest with yourself is extremely important for your success!

Weigh & measure self.

Date _____ Weight _____

Neck _____ Chin _____Bust_____ Mid____

Waist _____ Hips _____ Buttocks _____

R Arm __ L Arm__ R Thigh__ L Thigh __

R Knee ___L Knee ____

R Calf __ L Calf __R Ankle __ R Ankle __

Copy this into your journal; and take and record your measurements each week. You will love watching the numbers shrink. Weigh yourself and record it below; and each morning weigh in and record it in Phase Seven as well as in your journal.

Start drinking lemon water. Now! (lemon makes water more alkaline) and also helps you drink more of it.)

Get Honest with yourself. How is all this fat (there I said it) effecting you: Physically, emotionally spiritually, sexually, and yes financially.

Write it here: _____

_____

_____

_____

_____

_____

_____

_____

_____

_____

_____

_____

_____

_____

_____

_____

_____

_____

_____

_____

_____

_____

_____

_____

_____

_____

copy this to your journal and keep writing.

**PHASE TWO:**
**Journaling Yourself To Thin**
See Phase Seven for eating and activity journal. But in addition you will find a complete journal of your thoughts, feelings and activities very helpful. A simple notebook or a computer file will suffice, just start writing about feelings and you will be surprised how much you will learn about yourself; and how many issues you work out.

Journaling is the very best way to deal with old tapes and by writing you will journal Yourself Thin!

We've talked about old tapes. Well we didn't call them that- we called them emotions. Anytime an emotion is unrealistically strong or painful it is most assuredly an 'old tape'. You know those hurtful words someone yelled at you, names that you were called by some unkind or unthinking person. You have no doubt even repeated them yourself! You drop something and you call yourself dummy.... Or you over eat and you call yourself... well you get the idea. There is no tool that can help you deal with these old tapes like journaling. Through journaling you will be successful in Facing, Tracing, Erasing and then finally Replacing these old hurtful tapes. It will also help you identify people who are not helpful on your road to success, and help you work out ways to deal with them. You may see the need to eliminate a few hurtful people from your life. Humans are not a disposable commodity. We are enriched by the many different personalities we encounter and have around us. But occasionally there may be someone who is a real detriment to our emotional (and sometimes physical) health. But before deciding to disengage from a relationship no matter how close or distant, give it some good deep thought and then journal extensively about it,   Journaling will help you decide whether or not it would be a good choice for you. You may decide that just a short time and distance is necessary.  You may also realize that certain people are better friends than you realized. You will definitely find out through journaling that along with shedding baggage you will experience personal growth. Word of good advice- copy your notes on how you felt before, during and after eating along with who you ate with into your journal. You may see some emotional trends and be able to trace them to certain situations and/or person/persons.  It is well worth the effort to sort this stuff out!! As you figure out your triggers make sure to add them to your list in Tool #11.  And Hey! Reward yourself for taking the time and putting forth the effort

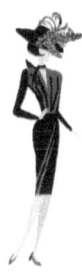

## FACE IT, TRACE IT, ERASE IT, REPLACE IT!

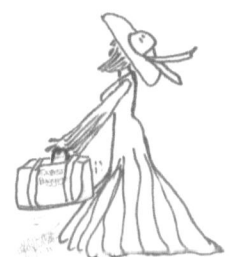

## PHASE THREE
MIND SET

This is an istance where the phrase "It's All In Your Head" is true.  You must have the right mind set to be successful on your plan.

The first section of this book has helped you start getting into a good frame of mind.  But you need more.  Gather and READ anything you've collected on weight loss REREAD  Gather more. (check library and book stores, magazine racks and the internet) Find photos and sayings to inspire you, and keep you motivated, print them out and frame or post them where you will see them often.  Writing them on the page designated for this purpose in the front of this book and keeping it in your pocket or bag for quick reference is also a good idea.  The time it takes to get into the proper and successful mind set is different for everyone.  You will know when you are ready.

## PHASE FOUR
YOUR PLAN

Choosing a healthy program that fits YOU. Don't call it that ugly four letter "d" word. Call it your plan or program or protocol- anything but 'diet'. And have a plan "B" incase you find your plan isn't working for you. You have so many to choose from... perhaps you've had limited success with a plan in the past, but just needed some tools to help you along. Maybe that would be a plan to try again. Whether it's 'Fit For Life, HTG, The Zone, or maybe you are prone to a Vegan way of eating- what ever you choose you should have the tools now to have success. Write Plan A & B in detail here:

_____

_____

_____

_____

_____

_____

_____

_____

_____

_____

_____

_____

_____

_____

_____

_____

_____

_____

_____

_____

_____

## PHASE FIVE
### Setting Goals & Rewards

There is much to be said for positive reinforcement! It's very important that you reward yourself. One thing that most of us have in common (other than the weight thing) is that we withhold good things from ourselves. (Giving your self/body harmful foods is not being good to your self.) In fact, you may even have difficulty choosing rewards for yourself. And it may take effort and practice to become comfortable with giving yourself good things. I've given you two ways to reward yourself. The first is for actions that will help you reach your goals, you'll earn points for these actions. You will cash these in for specific rewards. The second is for reaching those goals and you will be rewarded for each short and long term goal you reach. I've listed some activities that will earn you points; however YOU are in control of your plan. So I've added spaces for you to list some as well. YOU choose your goals and rewards.

### POINTS & REWARDS FOR DOIN' IT

You MUST reward yourself! And the rewards must be for YOU- after all it is YOU who earned them. For each 100 points you accumulate pick a reward from list below. 100 POINTS = (List rewards that you will spend these points, such as massage, pedi, mani, walk in favorite park)

_____

_____

_____

_____

_____

_____

_____

_____

_____

_____

Activities to earn points:

10 POINTS FOR: Starting DOIN' IT

Restarting DOIN' IT

Shopping instead of eating out

Choosing healthy meal  instead of junk

Snacking on Veggies, Fruit or Almonds

Dealing w/emotions instead of binging

EA 30 Min Card Stretches (see Phase 6)

EA 15-4-6 session (see last page)

Talking/Journaling About Anxiety
instead Of Binging

Walking 30 Min

EA 10 Min On Bike

EA 5 Min of Dancing

Taking Stairs Instead Of Elevator

Reading first part of this workbook

Re-reading first part of this workbook

Setting Short  & Long Term Goals

For Reaching Each Short
    Term Goal (earns double rewards)

For Reaching Long Term Goal(earns
    double rewards)

Now it's your turn to add some:

_____

_____

_____

_____

_____

_____

_____

_____

_____

_____

_____

_____

_____

_____

# Goals & Rewards

Start Date_____

Start Weight _____

Long Term Goal Weight _____

Long Term Reward _____

1st Short Term Goal _____

1$^{st}$ Short Term Reward _____

2$^{nd}$ Short Term Goal _____

2$^{nd}$ Short Term Reward _____

3$^{rd}$ Short Term Goal _____

3$^{rd}$ Short Term Reward _____

4$^{th}$ Short Term Goal _____

4$^{th}$ Short Term Reward _____

5$^{th}$ Short Term Goal _____

5$^{th}$ Short Term Reward _____

6$^{th}$ Short Term Goal _____

6$^{th}$ Short Term Reward _____

7$^{th}$ Short Term Goal __ _____

7$^{th}$ Short Term Reward _____

8$^{th}$ Short Term Goal _____

8$^{th}$ Short Term Reward _____

9$^{th}$ Short Term Goal _____

9$^{th}$ Short Term Reward _____

10$^{th}$ Short Term Goal _____

10$^{th}$ Short Term Reward _____

11$^{th}$ Short Term Goal _____

11$^{th}$ Short Term Reward _____

12$^{th}$ Short Term Goal _____

12$^{th}$ Short Term Reward _____

13$^{th}$ Short Term Goal _____

13$^{th}$ Short Term Reward _____

14$^{th}$ Short Term Goal _____

14$^{th}$ Short Term Reward _____

15$^{th}$ Short Term Goal _____

15$^{th}$ Short Term Reward _____

16$^{th}$ Short Term Goal _____

16$^{th}$ Short Term Reward _____

## PHASE SIX
Getting Active

Sit less, move more.  Humans were created with their own built in mode of transportation.  Use it.  Walk instead of driving when ever you can.  It's good for you and it's good for the environment. I've found that my body, after a year of suffering from an Achilles tendon and from doing not a whole lot outside of sitting at my computer and the occasional mad dash around the house tiding up, has become stiff and well this accompanied by my recent 62nd bd is not a welcome condition.  I've started tricking my body into doing stretches.

While watching some mindless 30 minute program on TV, I sit on floor with legs spread wide (or as wide as possible at this stage of the game) and play solitaire.  I deal the cards wide and far away so it is necessary to bend and stretch to reach them. I play game after game until program is over.  I shed an inch around my waist from this the first week.  And it's getting easier to get back up off the floor afterwards lol. It also worked to get me limbered up so I that I can move on to other activities. Like walking, dancing, biking, aerobics, gardening, and playing tennis,  ☺.

Choose fun activities you love to do and list below: (check with doctor before starting ):

_____
_____
_____
_____
_____
_____
_____
_____
_____
_____
_____

35

Before we move on to Phase Seven-
THE FOLLOWING BARES REPEATING:

**Give yourself the gift of your heart's desire-
Only <u>YOU</u> can make you thin.
NOTHING TASTES AS GOOD AS
HEALTHY, ENERGETIC & THIN FEELS
<u>And remember these important points:</u>**

- You have many feelings on many levels that will make unconscious choices *unless* you recognize them.
- To recognize feelings make a conscience effort to feel them. Keep a small pocket notebook with you at all times and every few moments jot down what you are feeling..... you will realize some feelings that have been 'installed' at different times in your life that may be inappropriate now. However until you deal with them they will continue to control your thoughts, actions and decisions and choices.
- **DON'T REACT....ACT**
    **Before making choices in life ask yourself:**
1. **What will this choice produce?**

                                        **and**
2. **Am I willing and ready to accept the consequences (with out thinking I can control or change them)?**


Congratulations! You are now ready to start DOIN' IT!

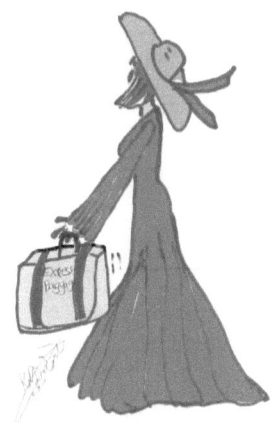

## PHASE SEVEN
### Doin' It

Record today's date, your weight and measurements here(copy them to your journal as well): Put today's date even though you haven't began the 'Doin' It' plan yet. Well actually you have. You've started Phase three. If it's been a week since you measured yourself measure again. And don't forget to transcribe the results into your journal.

Date _____ Weight _____

Neck _____ Chin _____Bust_____ Mid____

Waist _____ Hips _____ Buttocks _____

R Arm __L Arm__ R Thigh__ L Thigh __

R Knee ___L Knee ____

R Calf __ L Calf __R Ankle __ R Ankle __

## Eating & Activity Journal

Keep track of daily Food & Water intake, Feelings, Emotions, People, Exercise. Along with writing feelings, draw a happy/sad/angry/etc face to describe feelings. Experts say you should drink 1/3 – 1/2 oz of water for each pound you weigh . Keep track of water intake. Check with doctor before starting any exercise or weight loss program.

## DAY ONE Date_____ Weight_____

Oz of Lemon Water drank today _____

Breakfast: _____

Who I ate with: _____

How I felt before/during/after I ate: _____

_____

Snack:_____

Who I ate with: _____

How I felt before/during/after I ate: _____

_____

Lunch: _____

Who I ate with: _____

How I felt before/during/after I ate: _____

_____

Snack _____

Who I ate with: _____

How I felt before/during/after I ate: _____

_____

Dinner: _____

Who I ate with: _____

How I felt before/during/after I ate: _____

_____

_____

Snack:_____

Who I ate with: _____

How I felt before/during/after I ate: _____

_____

What I did today that counts as exercise (in addition to my daily activities) include how long: _____

_____

**DAY TWO Date_____Weight_____**

Oz of Lemon Water drank today _____

Breakfast: _____

Who I ate with: _____

How I felt before/during/after I ate: _____

_____

Snack:_____

Who I ate with: _____

How I felt before/during/after I ate: _____

_____

Lunch: _____

Who I ate with: _____

How I felt before/during/after I ate: _____

_____

Snack _____

Who I ate with: _____

How I felt before/during/after I ate: _____

_____

Dinner: _____

Who I ate with: _____

How I felt before/during/after I ate: _____

_____

_____

Snack:_____

Who I ate with: _____

How I felt before/during/after I ate: _____

_____

What I did today that counts as exercise (in addition to my daily
activities) include how long: _____

_____

**DAY THREE  Date**_____ **Weight**_____

Oz of  Lemon Water drank today _____

Breakfast: _____

Who I ate with: _____

How I felt before/during/after I ate: _____

_____

Snack:_____

Who I ate with: _____

How I felt before/during/after I ate: _____

_____

Lunch: _____

Who I ate with: _____

How I felt before/during/after I ate: _____

_____

Snack _____

Who I ate with: _____

How I felt before/during/after I ate: _____

_____

Dinner: _____

Who I ate with: _____

How I felt before/during/after I ate: _____

_____

_____

Snack:_____

Who I ate with: _____

How I felt before/during/after I ate: _____

_____

What I did today that counts as exercise (in addition to my daily

activities) include how long: _____

_____

**DAY FOUR Date_____ Weight_____**

Oz of Lemon Water drank today _____

Breakfast: _____

Who I ate with: _____

How I felt before/during/after I ate: _____

_____

Snack:_____

Who I ate with: _____

How I felt before/during/after I ate: _____

_____

Lunch: _____

Who I ate with: _____

How I felt before/during/after I ate: _____

_____

Snack _____

Who I ate with: _____

How I felt before/during/after I ate: _____

_____

Dinner: _____

Who I ate with: _____

How I felt before/during/after I ate: _____

_____

_____

Snack:_____

Who I ate with: _____

How I felt before/during/after I ate: _____

_____

What I did today that counts as exercise (in addition to my daily
activities) include how long: _____

_____

## DAY FIVE  Date_____  Weight_____

Oz of  Lemon Water drank today  _____

Breakfast: _____

Who I ate with: _____

How I felt before/during/after I ate: _____

_____

Snack:_____

Who I ate with: _____

How I felt before/during/after I ate: _____

_____

Lunch: _____

Who I ate with: _____

How I felt before/during/after I ate: _____

_____

Snack _____

Who I ate with: _____

How I felt before/during/after I ate: _____

_____

Dinner: _____

Who I ate with: _____

How I felt before/during/after I ate: _____

_____

_____

Snack:_____

Who I ate with: _____

How I felt before/during/after I ate: _____

_____

What I did today that counts as exercise (in addition to my daily
activities) include how long: _____

_____

**DAY SIX  Date_____  Weight_____**

Oz of  Lemon Water drank today _____

Breakfast: _____

Who I ate with: _____

How I felt before/during/after I ate: _____

_____

Snack:_____

Who I ate with: _____

How I felt before/during/after I ate: _____

_____

Lunch: _____

Who I ate with: _____

How I felt before/during/after I ate: _____

_____

Snack _____

Who I ate with: _____

How I felt before/during/after I ate: _____

_____

Dinner: _____

Who I ate with: _____

How I felt before/during/after I ate: _____

_____

_____

Snack:_____

Who I ate with: _____

How I felt before/during/after I ate: _____

_____

What I did today that counts as exercise (in addition to my daily

activities) include how long: _____

_____

**DAY SEVEN  Date_____Weight_____**

Oz of  Lemon Water drank today _____

Breakfast: _____

Who I ate with: _____

How I felt before/during/after I ate: _____

_____

Snack:_____

Who I ate with: _____

How I felt before/during/after I ate: _____

_____

Lunch: _____

Who I ate with: _____

How I felt before/during/after I ate: _____

_____

Snack _____

Who I ate with: _____

How I felt before/during/after I ate: _____

_____

Dinner: _____

Who I ate with: _____

How I felt before/during/after I ate: _____

_____

_____

Snack:_____

Who I ate with: _____

How I felt before/during/after I ate: _____

_____

What I did today that counts as exercise (in addition to my daily
activities) include how long: _____

_____

## DAY EIGHT  Date _____   Weight _____

Oz of  Lemon Water drank today _____

Breakfast: _____

Who I ate with: _____

How I felt before/during/after I ate: _____

_____

Snack:_____

Who I ate with: _____

How I felt before/during/after I ate: _____

_____

Lunch: _____

Who I ate with: _____

How I felt before/during/after I ate: _____

_____

Snack _____

Who I ate with: _____

How I felt before/during/after I ate: _____

_____

Dinner: _____

Who I ate with: _____

How I felt before/during/after I ate: _____

_____

_____

Snack:_____

Who I ate with: _____

How I felt before/during/after I ate: _____

_____

What I did today that counts as exercise (in addition to my daily

activities) include how long: _____

_____

## DAY  NINE     Date _____ Weight _____

Oz of Lemon Water drank today _____

Breakfast: _____

Who I ate with: _____

How I felt before/during/after I ate: _____

_____

Snack:_____

Who I ate with: _____

How I felt before/during/after I ate: _____

_____

Lunch: _____

Who I ate with: _____

How I felt before/during/after I ate: _____

_____

Snack _____

Who I ate with: _____

How I felt before/during/after I ate: _____

_____

Dinner: _____

Who I ate with: _____

How I felt before/during/after I ate: _____

_____

_____

Snack:_____

Who I ate with: _____

How I felt before/during/after I ate: _____

_____

What I did today that counts as exercise (in addition to my daily

activities) include how long: _____

_____

**DAY TEN Date** _____ **Weight** _____

Oz of Lemon Water drank today _____

Breakfast: _____

Who I ate with: _____

How I felt before/during/after I ate: _____

_____

Snack: _____

Who I ate with: _____

How I felt before/during/after I ate: _____

_____

Lunch: _____

Who I ate with: _____

How I felt before/during/after I ate: _____

_____

Snack _____

Who I ate with: _____

How I felt before/during/after I ate: _____

_____

Dinner: _____

Who I ate with: _____

IIow I felt before/during/after I ate: _____

_____

_____

Snack: _____

Who I ate with: _____

How I felt before/during/after I ate: _____

_____

What I did today that counts as exercise (in addition to my daily

activities) include how long: _____

_____

47

**DAY ELEVEN  Date** _____ **Weight** _____

Oz of  Lemon Water drank today  _____

Breakfast: _____

Who I ate with: _____

How I felt before/during/after I ate: _____

_____

Snack:_____

Who I ate with: _____

How I felt before/during/after I ate: _____

_____

Lunch: _____

Who I ate with: _____

How I felt before/during/after I ate: _____

_____

Snack _____

Who I ate with: _____

How I felt before/during/after I ate: _____

_____

Dinner: _____

Who I ate with: _____

How I felt before/during/after I ate: _____

_____

_____

Snack:_____

Who I ate with: _____

How I felt before/during/after I ate: _____

_____

What I did today that counts as exercise (in addition to my daily

activities) include how long: _____

_____

**DAY TWELVE  Date_____ Weight_____**

Oz of  Lemon Water drank today _____

Breakfast: _____

Who I ate with: _____

How I felt before/during/after I ate: _____

_____

Snack:_____

Who I ate with: _____

How I felt before/during/after I ate: _____

_____

Lunch: _____

Who I ate with: _____

How I felt before/during/after I ate: _____

_____

Snack _____

Who I ate with: _____

How I felt before/during/after I ate: _____

_____

Dinner: _____

Who I ate with: _____

How I felt before/during/after I ate: _____

_____

_____

Snack:_____

Who I ate with: _____

How I felt before/during/after I ate: _____

_____

What I did today that counts as exercise (in addition to my daily

activities) include how long: _____

_____

**DAY THIRTEEN  Date** _____ **Weight** _____

Oz of Lemon Water drank today _____

Breakfast: _____

Who I ate with: _____

How I felt before/during/after I ate: _____

_____

Snack:_____

Who I ate with: _____

How I felt before/during/after I ate: _____

_____

Lunch: _____

Who I ate with: _____

How I felt before/during/after I ate: _____

_____

Snack _____

Who I ate with: _____

How I felt before/during/after I ate: _____

_____

Dinner: _____

Who I ate with: _____

How I felt before/during/after I ate: _____

_____

_____

Snack:_____

Who I ate with: _____

How I felt before/during/after I ate: _____

_____

What I did today that counts as exercise (in addition to my daily
activities) include how long: _____

_____

**DAY FOURTEEN  Date_____  Weight_____**

Oz of Lemon Water drank today _____

Breakfast: _____

Who I ate with: _____

How I felt before/during/after I ate: _____

_____

Snack:_____

Who I ate with: _____

How I felt before/during/after I ate: _____

_____

Lunch: _____

Who I ate with: _____

How I felt before/during/after I ate: _____

_____

Snack _____

Who I ate with: _____

How I felt before/during/after I ate: _____

_____

Dinner: _____

Who I ate with: _____

How I felt before/during/after I ate: _____

_____

_____

Snack:_____

Who I ate with: _____

How I felt before/during/after I ate: _____

_____

What I did today that counts as exercise (in addition to my daily

activities) include how long: _____

_____

## DAY FIFTEEN   Date _____   Weight _____

Oz of  Lemon Water drank today _____

Breakfast: _____

Who I ate with: _____

How I felt before/during/after I ate: _____

_____

Snack:_____

Who I ate with: _____

How I felt before/during/after I ate: _____

_____

Lunch: _____

Who I ate with: _____

How I felt before/during/after I ate: _____

_____

Snack _____

Who I ate with: _____

How I felt before/during/after I ate: _____

_____

Dinner: _____

Who I ate with: _____

How I felt before/during/after I ate: _____

_____

_____

Snack:_____

Who I ate with: _____

How I felt before/during/after I ate: _____

_____

What I did today that counts as exercise (in addition to my daily

activities) include how long: _____

_____

## DAY SIXTEEN  Date _____ Weight _____

Oz of Lemon Water drank today _____

Breakfast: _____

Who I ate with: _____

How I felt before/during/after I ate: _____

_____

Snack: _____

Who I ate with: _____

How I felt before/during/after I ate: _____

_____

Lunch: _____

Who I ate with: _____

How I felt before/during/after I ate: _____

_____

Snack _____

Who I ate with: _____

How I felt before/during/after I ate: _____

_____

Dinner: _____

Who I ate with: _____

How I felt before/during/after I ate: _____

_____

_____

Snack: _____

Who I ate with: _____

How I felt before/during/after I ate: _____

_____

What I did today that counts as exercise (in addition to my daily

activities) include how long: _____

_____

53

## DAY SEVENTEEN   Date_____ Weight_____

Oz of Lemon Water drank today _____

Breakfast: _____

Who I ate with: _____

How I felt before/during/after I ate: _____

_____

Snack:_____

Who I ate with: _____

How I felt before/during/after I ate: _____

_____

Lunch: _____

Who I ate with: _____

How I felt before/during/after I ate: _____

_____

Snack _____

Who I ate with: _____

How I felt before/during/after I ate: _____

_____

Dinner: _____

Who I ate with: _____

How I felt before/during/after I ate: _____

_____

_____

Snack:_____

Who I ate with: _____

How I felt before/during/after I ate: _____

_____

What I did today that counts as exercise (in addition to my daily
activities) include how long: _____

_____

**DAY 18    Date_____    Weight_____**

Oz of  Lemon Water drank today _____

Breakfast: _____

Who I ate with: _____

How I felt before/during/after I ate: _____

_____

Snack:_____

Who I ate with: _____

How I felt before/during/after I ate: _____

_____

Lunch: _____

Who I ate with: _____

How I felt before/during/after I ate: _____

_____

Snack _____

Who I ate with: _____

How I felt before/during/after I ate: _____

_____

Dinner: _____

Who I ate with: _____

How I felt before/during/after I ate: _____    _____

_____

_____

Snack:_____

Who I ate with: _____

How I felt before/during/after I ate: _____

_____

What I did today that counts as exercise (in addition to my daily

activities) include how long: _____

_____

## DAY 19  Date_____ Weight_____

Oz of Lemon Water drank today _____

Breakfast: _____

Who I ate with: _____

How I felt before/during/after I ate: _____
_____

Snack:_____

Who I ate with: _____

How I felt before/during/after I ate: _____
_____

Lunch: _____

Who I ate with: _____

How I felt before/during/after I ate: _____
_____

Snack _____

Who I ate with: _____

How I felt before/during/after I ate: _____
_____

Dinner: _____

Who I ate with: _____

How I felt before/during/after I ate: _____
_____
_____

Snack:_____

Who I ate with: _____

How I felt before/during/after I ate: _____
_____

What I did today that counts as exercise (in addition to my daily
activities) include how long: _____
_____

**DAY 20 Date_____ Weight_____**

Oz of Lemon Water drank today _____

Breakfast: _____

Who I ate with: _____

How I felt before/during/after I ate: _____

_____

Snack:_____

Who I ate with: _____

How I felt before/during/after I ate: _____

_____

Lunch: _____

Who I ate with: _____

How I felt before/during/after I ate: _____

_____

Snack _____

Who I ate with: _____

How I felt before/during/after I ate: _____

_____

Dinner: _____

Who I ate with: _____

How I felt before/during/after I ate: _____

_____

_____

Snack:_____

Who I ate with: _____

How I felt before/during/after I ate: _____

_____

What I did today that counts as exercise (in addition to my daily

activities) include how long: _____

_____

## DAY 21 Date_____ Weight_____

Oz of Lemon Water drank today _____

Breakfast: _____

Who I ate with: _____

How I felt before/during/after I ate: _____

_____

Snack:_____

Who I ate with: _____

How I felt before/during/after I ate: _____

_____

Lunch: _____

Who I ate with: _____

How I felt before/during/after I ate: _____

_____

Snack _____

Who I ate with: _____

How I felt before/during/after I ate: _____

_____

Dinner: _____

Who I ate with: _____

How I felt before/during/after I ate: _____

_____

_____

Snack:_____

Who I ate with: _____

How I felt before/during/after I ate: _____

_____

What I did today that counts as exercise (in addition to my daily
activities) include how long: _____

_____

## DAY 22 Date_____ Weight_____

Oz of Lemon Water drank today _____

Breakfast: _____

Who I ate with: _____

How I felt before/during/after I ate: _____

_____

Snack:_____

Who I ate with: _____

How I felt before/during/after I ate: _____

_____

Lunch: _____

Who I ate with: _____

How I felt before/during/after I ate: _____

_____

Snack _____

Who I ate with: _____

How I felt before/during/after I ate: _____

_____

Dinner: _____

Who I ate with: _____

How I felt before/during/after I ate: ___ _____

_____

_____

Snack:_____

Who I ate with: _____

How I felt before/during/after I ate: _____

_____

What I did today that counts as exercise (in addition to my daily
activities) include how long: _____

_____

**DAY 23  Date_____ Weight_____**

Oz of Lemon Water drank today _____

Breakfast: _____

Who I ate with: _____

How I felt before/during/after I ate: _____

_____

Snack:_____

Who I ate with: _____

How I felt before/during/after I ate: _____

_____

Lunch: _____

Who I ate with: _____

How I felt before/during/after I ate: _____

_____

Snack _____

Who I ate with: _____

How I felt before/during/after I ate: _____

_____

Dinner: _____

Who I ate with: _____

How I felt before/during/after I ate: _____

_____

_____

Snack:_____

Who I ate with: _____

How I felt before/during/after I ate: _____

_____

What I did today that counts as exercise (in addition to my daily
activities) include how long: _____

_____

## DAY  24  Date_____ Weight_____

Oz of Lemon Water drank today _____

Breakfast: _____

Who I ate with: _____

How I felt before/during/after I ate: _____

_____

Snack:_____

Who I ate with: _____

How I felt before/during/after I ate: _____

_____

Lunch: _____

Who I ate with: _____

How I felt before/during/after I ate: _____

_____

Snack _____

Who I ate with: _____

How I felt before/during/after I ate: _____

_____

Dinner: _____

Who I ate with: _____

How I felt before/during/after I ate: _____

_____

_____

Snack:_____

Who I ate with: _____

How I felt before/during/after I ate: _____

_____

What I did today that counts as exercise (in addition to my daily
activities) include how long: _____

_____

61

## DAY  25  Date_____ Weight_____

Oz of  Lemon Water drank today _____

Breakfast: _____

Who I ate with: _____

How I felt before/during/after I ate: _____

_____

Snack:_____

Who I ate with: _____

How I felt before/during/after I ate: _____

_____

Lunch: _____

Who I ate with: _____

How I felt before/during/after I ate: _____

_____

Snack _____

Who I ate with: _____

How I felt before/during/after I ate: _____

_____

Dinner: _____

Who I ate with: _____

How I felt before/during/after I ate: _____

_____

_____

Snack:_____

Who I ate with: _____

How I felt before/during/after I ate: _____

_____

What I did today that counts as exercise (in addition to my daily
activities) include how long: _____

_____

## DAY 26  Date_____ Weight_____

Oz of  Lemon Water drank today _____

Breakfast: _____

Who I ate with: _____

How I felt before/during/after I ate: _____

_____

Snack:_____

Who I ate with: _____

How I felt before/during/after I ate: _____

_____

Lunch: _____

Who I ate with: _____

How I felt before/during/after I ate: _____

_____

Snack _____

Who I ate with: _____

How I felt before/during/after I ate: _____

_____

Dinner: _____

Who I ate with: _____

How I felt before/during/after I ate: _____

_____

_____

Snack:_____

Who I ate with: _____

How I felt before/during/after I ate: _____

_____

What I did today that counts as exercise (in addition to my daily

activities) include how long: _____

_____

63

**DAY 27    Date_____Weight_____**

Oz of Lemon Water drank today _____

Breakfast: _____

Who I ate with: _____

How I felt before/during/after I ate: _____

_____

Snack:_____

Who I ate with: _____

How I felt before/during/after I ate: _____

_____

Lunch: _____

Who I ate with: _____

How I felt before/during/after I ate: _____

_____

Snack _____

Who I ate with: _____

How I felt before/during/after I ate: _____

_____

Dinner: _____

Who I ate with: _____

How I felt before/during/after I ate: _____

_____

_____

Snack:_____

Who I ate with: _____

How I felt before/during/after I ate: _____

_____

What I did today that counts as exercise (in addition to my daily
activities) include how long: _____

_____

## DAY 28   Date _____   Weight _____

Oz of Lemon Water drank today _____

Breakfast: _____

Who I ate with: _____

How I felt before/during/after I ate: _____

_____

Snack: _____

Who I ate with: _____

How I felt before/during/after I ate: _____

_____

Lunch: _____

Who I ate with: _____

How I felt before/during/after I ate: _____

_____

Snack _____

Who I ate with: _____

How I felt before/during/after I ate: _____

_____

Dinner: _____

Who I ate with: _____

How I felt before/during/after I ate: _____

_____

_____

Snack: _____

Who I ate with: _____

How I felt before/during/after I ate: _____

_____

What I did today that counts as exercise (in addition to my daily

activities) include how long: _____

_____

## DAY  29    Date_____    Weight_____

Oz of  Lemon Water drank today _____

Breakfast: _____

Who I ate with: _____

How I felt before/during/after I ate: _____

_____

Snack:_____

Who I ate with: _____

How I felt before/during/after I ate: _____

_____

Lunch: _____

Who I ate with: _____

How I felt before/during/after I ate: _____

_____

Snack _____

Who I ate with: _____

How I felt before/during/after I ate: _____

_____

Dinner: _____

Who I ate with: _____

How I felt before/during/after I ate: _____

_____

_____

Snack:_____

Who I ate with: _____

How I felt before/during/after I ate: _____

_____

What I did today that counts as exercise (in addition to my daily
activities) include how long: _____

_____

## DAY 30   Date_____   Weight_____

Oz of Lemon Water drank today _____

Breakfast: _____

Who I ate with: _____

How I felt before/during/after I ate: _____

_____

Snack:_____

Who I ate with: _____

How I felt before/during/after I ate: _____

_____

Lunch: _____

Who I ate with: _____

How I felt before/during/after I ate: _____

_____

Snack _____

Who I ate with: _____

How I felt before/during/after I ate: _____

_____

Dinner: _____

Who I ate with: _____

How I felt before/during/after I ate: _____

_____

_____

Snack:_____

Who I ate with: _____

How I felt before/during/after I ate: _____

_____

What I did today that counts as exercise (in addition to my daily
activities) include how long: _____

_____

67

## DAY 31    Date _____    Weight _____

Oz of Lemon Water drank today _____

Breakfast: _____

Who I ate with: _____

How I felt before/during/after I ate: _____
_____

Snack:_____

Who I ate with: _____

How I felt before/during/after I ate: _____
_____

Lunch: _____

Who I ate with: _____

How I felt before/during/after I ate: _____
_____

Snack _____

Who I ate with: _____

How I felt before/during/after I ate: _____
_____

Dinner: _____

Who I ate with: _____

How I felt before/during/after I ate: _____
_____
_____

Snack:_____

Who I ate with: _____

How I felt before/during/after I ate: _____
_____

What I did today that counts as exercise (in addition to my daily activities) include how long: _____
_____

CONGRATULATIONS!  You've been Doin' It for ONE Month!  Reward Yourself!!

If you haven't reached half way to your Long Term Goal Order another workbook to be prepared to continue

DOIN' IT!

And if this is your  $2^{nd}$  (or $3^{rd}$) time around Congratulations on your tenacity!!  REWARD YOURSELF!

If you HAVE reached your goal- Congratulations and enjoy your reward!!

Keep this book as a keepsake of your road to success!  Read your inspirational thoughts often!

Don't forget all the things you've learned about yourself.

Keep your 'Tool Box' handy and watch out for those Triggering Situations and Events.

Stay connected to your Support Team and any online or group supports that you've connected with.  Beware of the 'false friends' who would love nothing better than to bully you back into the mold where THEY were comfortable having you.  Remember you've done this for yourself!

You Deserve to be Fit, Healthy & Thin & Strong!

If you catch yourself gathering any more excess baggage whether in the form of old tapes or fat take a breath and

JUST LET GO!

You may also enjoy 15-4 6  by Kit DeCanti which is 'No Sweat' exercise routine which she developed and put on CD and DVD.  Check out her website for more information.

http://www.kitdeeproductions.com

**DAY  32**          **Date**                    **Weight**

Oz of  Lemon Water drank today _____

Breakfast: _____

Who I ate with: _____

How I felt before/during/after I ate: _____

_____

Snack:_____

Who I ate with: _____

How I felt before/during/after I ate: _____

_____

Lunch: _____

Who I ate with: _____

How I felt before/during/after I ate: _____

_____

Snack _____

Who I ate with: _____

How I felt before/during/after I ate: _____

_____

Dinner: _____

Who I ate with: _____

How I felt before/during/after I ate: _____

_____

_____

Snack:_____

Who I ate with: _____

How I felt before/during/after I ate: _____

_____

What I did today that counts as exercise (in addition to my daily

activities) include how long: _____

_____

**DAY  33____Date_____Weight_____**

Oz of  Lemon Water drank today _____

Breakfast: _____

Who I ate with: _____

How I felt before/during/after I ate: _____

_____

Snack:_____

Who I ate with: _____

How I felt before/during/after I ate: _____

_____

Lunch: _____

Who I ate with: _____

How I felt before/during/after I ate: _____

_____

Snack _____

Who I ate with: _____

How I felt before/during/after I ate: _____

_____

Dinner: _____

Who I ate with: _____

How I felt before/during/after I ate: _____

_____

_____

Snack:_____

Who I ate with: _____

How I felt before/during/after I ate: _____

_____

What I did today that counts as exercise (in addition to my daily

activities) include how long: _____

_____

**DAY  34**       **Date**          **Weight**

Oz of  Lemon Water drank today _____

Breakfast: _____

Who I ate with: _____

How I felt before/during/after I ate: _____

_____

Snack:_____

Who I ate with: _____

How I felt before/during/after I ate: _____

_____

Lunch: _____

Who I ate with: _____

How I felt before/during/after I ate: _____

_____

Snack _____

Who I ate with: _____

How I felt before/during/after I ate: _____

_____

Dinner: _____

Who I ate with: _____

How I felt before/during/after I ate: _____

_____

_____

Snack:_____

Who I ate with: _____

How I felt before/during/after I ate: _____

_____

What I did today that counts as exercise (in addition to my daily
activities) include how long: _____

_____

**DAY  35        Date            Weight_____**

Oz of  Lemon Water drank today _____

Breakfast: _____

Who I ate with: _____

How I felt before/during/after I ate: _____

_____

Snack:_____

Who I ate with: _____

How I felt before/during/after I ate: _____

_____

Lunch: _____

Who I ate with: _____

How I felt before/during/after I ate: _____

_____

Snack _____

Who I ate with: _____

How I felt before/during/after I ate: _____

_____

Dinner: _____

Who I ate with: _____

How I felt before/during/after I ate: _____

_____

_____

Snack:_____

Who I ate with: _____

How I felt before/during/after I ate: _____

_____

What I did today that counts as exercise (in addition to my daily

activities) include how long: _____

_____

## DAY 36  Date_____ Weight_____

Oz of Lemon Water drank today _____

Breakfast: _____

Who I ate with: _____

How I felt before/during/after I ate: _____
_____

Snack:_____

Who I ate with: _____

How I felt before/during/after I ate: _____
_____

Lunch: _____

Who I ate with: _____

How I felt before/during/after I ate: _____
_____

Snack _____

Who I ate with: _____

How I felt before/during/after I ate: _____
_____

Dinner: _____

Who I ate with: _____

How I felt before/during/after I ate: _____
_____
_____

Snack:_____

Who I ate with: _____

How I felt before/during/after I ate: _____
_____

What I did today that counts as exercise (in addition to my daily activities) include how long: _____
_____

## DAY 37  Date_____  Weight_____

Oz of Lemon Water drank today _____

Breakfast: _____

Who I ate with: _____

How I felt before/during/after I ate: _____

_____

Snack:_____

Who I ate with: _____

How I felt before/during/after I ate: _____

_____

Lunch: _____

Who I ate with: _____

How I felt before/during/after I ate: _____

_____

Snack _____

Who I ate with: _____

How I felt before/during/after I ate: _____

_____

Dinner: _____

Who I ate with: _____

How I felt before/during/after I ate: _____

_____

_____

Snack:_____

Who I ate with: _____

How I felt before/during/after I ate: _____

_____

What I did today that counts as exercise (in addition to my daily

activities) include how long: _____

_____

75

## DAY 38  Date_____  Weight_____

Oz of Lemon Water drank today _____

Breakfast: _____

Who I ate with: _____

How I felt before/during/after I ate: _____

_____

Snack:_____

Who I ate with: _____

How I felt before/during/after I ate: _____

_____

Lunch: _____

Who I ate with: _____

How I felt before/during/after I ate: _____

_____

Snack _____

Who I ate with: _____

How I felt before/during/after I ate: _____

_____

Dinner: _____

Who I ate with: _____

How I felt before/during/after I ate: _____

_____

_____

Snack:_____

Who I ate with: _____

How I felt before/during/after I ate: _____

_____

What I did today that counts as exercise (in addition to my daily

activities) include how long: _____

_____

**DAY 39  Date_____  Weight_____**

Oz of Lemon Water drank today _____

Breakfast: _____

Who I ate with: _____

How I felt before/during/after I ate: _____

_____

Snack:_____

Who I ate with: _____

How I felt before/during/after I ate: _____

_____

Lunch: _____

Who I ate with: _____

How I felt before/during/after I ate: _____

_____

Snack _____

Who I ate with: _____

How I felt before/during/after I ate: _____

_____

Dinner: _____

Who I ate with: _____

How I felt before/during/after I ate: _____

_____

_____

Snack:_____

Who I ate with: _____

How I felt before/during/after I ate: _____

_____

What I did today that counts as exercise (in addition to my daily

activities) include how long: _____

_____

**DAY  40      Date_____  Weight_____**

Oz of  Lemon Water drank today _____

Breakfast: _____

Who I ate with: _____

How I felt before/during/after I ate: _____

_____

Snack:_____

Who I ate with: _____

How I felt before/during/after I ate: _____

_____

Lunch: _____

Who I ate with: _____

How I felt before/during/after I ate: _____

_____

Snack _____

Who I ate with: _____

How I felt before/during/after I ate: _____

_____

Dinner: _____

Who I ate with: _____

How I felt before/during/after I ate: _____

_____

_____

Snack:_____

Who I ate with: _____

How I felt before/during/after I ate: _____

_____

What I did today that counts as exercise (in addition to my daily
activities) include how long: _____

_____

**DAY  41  Date_____Weight_____**

Oz of Lemon Water drank today _____

Breakfast: _____

Who I ate with: _____

How I felt before/during/after I ate: _____

_____

Snack:_____

Who I ate with: _____

How I felt before/during/after I ate: _____

_____

Lunch: _____

Who I ate with: _____

How I felt before/during/after I ate: _____

_____

Snack _____

Who I ate with: _____

How I felt before/during/after I ate: _____

_____

Dinner: _____

Who I ate with: _____

How I felt before/during/after I ate: _____

_____

_____

Snack:_____

Who I ate with: _____

How I felt before/during/after I ate: _____

_____

What I did today that counts as exercise (in addition to my daily
activities) include how long: _____

_____

**DAY 42   Date_____   Weight_____**

Oz of  Lemon Water drank today _____

Breakfast: _____

Who I ate with: _____

How I felt before/during/after I ate: _____

_____

Snack:_____

Who I ate with: _____

How I felt before/during/after I ate: _____

_____

Lunch: _____

Who I ate with: _____

How I felt before/during/after I ate: _____

_____

Snack _____

Who I ate with: _____

How I felt before/during/after I ate: _____

_____

Dinner: _____

Who I ate with: _____

How I felt before/during/after I ate: _____

_____

_____

Snack:_____

Who I ate with: _____

How I felt before/during/after I ate: _____

_____

What I did today that counts as exercise (in addition to my daily

activities) include how long: _____

_____

**DAY 43  Date _____ Weight _____**

Oz of Lemon Water drank today _____

Breakfast: _____

Who I ate with: _____

How I felt before/during/after I ate: _____

_____

Snack:_____

Who I ate with: _____

How I felt before/during/after I ate: _____

_____

Lunch: _____

Who I ate with: _____

How I felt before/during/after I ate: _____

_____

Snack _____

Who I ate with: _____

How I felt before/during/after I ate: _____

_____

Dinner: _____

Who I ate with: _____

How I felt before/during/after I ate: _____

_____

_____

Snack:_____

Who I ate with: _____

How I felt before/during/after I ate: _____

_____

What I did today that counts as exercise (in addition to my daily

activities) include how long: _____

_____

## DAY 44   Date_____   Weight_____

Oz of  Lemon Water drank today _____

Breakfast: _____

Who I ate with: _____

How I felt before/during/after I ate: _____

_____

Snack:_____

Who I ate with: _____

How I felt before/during/after I ate: _____

_____

Lunch: _____

Who I ate with: _____

How I felt before/during/after I ate: _____

_____

Snack _____

Who I ate with: _____

How I felt before/during/after I ate: _____

_____

Dinner: _____

Who I ate with: _____

How I felt before/during/after I ate: _____

_____

_____

Snack:_____

Who I ate with: _____

How I felt before/during/after I ate: _____

_____

What I did today that counts as exercise (in addition to my daily

activities) include how long: _____

_____

## DAY 45  Date_____ Weight_____

Oz of Lemon Water drank today _____

Breakfast: _____

Who I ate with: _____

How I felt before/during/after I ate: _____

_____

Snack:_____

Who I ate with: _____

How I felt before/during/after I ate: _____

_____

Lunch: _____

Who I ate with: _____

How I felt before/during/after I ate: _____

_____

Snack _____

Who I ate with: _____

How I felt before/during/after I ate: _____

_____

Dinner: _____

Who I ate with: _____

How I felt before/during/after I ate: _____

_____

_____

Snack:_____

Who I ate with: _____

How I felt before/during/after I ate: _____

_____

What I did today that counts as exercise (in addition to my daily

activities) include how long: _____

_____

## DAY 46  Date_____  Weight_____

Oz of Lemon Water drank today _____

Breakfast: _____

Who I ate with: _____

How I felt before/during/after I ate: _____

_____

Snack:_____

Who I ate with: _____

How I felt before/during/after I ate: _____

_____

Lunch: _____

Who I ate with: _____

How I felt before/during/after I ate: _____

_____

Snack _____

Who I ate with: _____

How I felt before/during/after I ate: _____

_____

Dinner: _____

Who I ate with: _____

How I felt before/during/after I ate: _____

_____

_____

Snack:_____

Who I ate with: _____

How I felt before/during/after I ate: _____

_____

What I did today that counts as exercise (in addition to my daily
activities) include how long: _____

_____

**DAY47_____ Date_____ Weight_____**

Oz of Lemon Water drank today _____

Breakfast: _____

Who I ate with: _____

How I felt before/during/after I ate: _____

_____

Snack:_____

Who I ate with: _____

How I felt before/during/after I ate: _____

_____

Lunch: _____

Who I ate with: _____

How I felt before/during/after I ate: _____

_____

Snack _____

Who I ate with: _____

How I felt before/during/after I ate: _____

_____

Dinner: _____

Who I ate with: _____

How I felt before/during/after I ate: _____

_____

_____

Snack:_____

Who I ate with: _____

How I felt before/during/after I ate: _____

_____

What I did today that counts as exercise (in addition to my daily

activities) include how long: _____

_____

## DAY 48  Date_____ Weight____

Oz of Lemon Water drank today _____

Breakfast: _____

Who I ate with: _____

How I felt before/during/after I ate: _____

_____

Snack:_____

Who I ate with: _____

How I felt before/during/after I ate: _____

_____

Lunch: _____

Who I ate with: _____

How I felt before/during/after I ate: _____

_____

Snack _____

Who I ate with: _____

How I felt before/during/after I ate: _____

_____

Dinner: _____

Who I ate with: _____

How I felt before/during/after I ate: _____

_____

_____

Snack:_____

Who I ate with: _____

How I felt before/during/after I ate: _____

_____

What I did today that counts as exercise (in addition to my daily
activities) include how long: _____

_____

## DAY 49   Date_____   Weight_____

Oz of Lemon Water drank today _____

Breakfast: _____

Who I ate with: _____

How I felt before/during/after I ate: _____

_____

Snack:_____

Who I ate with: _____

How I felt before/during/after I ate: _____

_____

Lunch: _____

Who I ate with: _____

How I felt before/during/after I ate: _____

_____

Snack _____

Who I ate with: _____

How I felt before/during/after I ate: _____

_____

Dinner: _____

Who I ate with: _____

How I felt before/during/after I ate: _____

_____

_____

Snack:_____

Who I ate with: _____

How I felt before/during/after I ate: _____

_____

What I did today that counts as exercise (in addition to my daily

activities) include how long: _____

_____

**DAY 50 Date_____ Weight_____**

Oz of Lemon Water drank today _____

Breakfast: _____

Who I ate with: _____

How I felt before/during/after I ate: _____

_____

Snack:_____

Who I ate with: _____

How I felt before/during/after I ate: _____

_____

Lunch: _____

Who I ate with: _____

How I felt before/during/after I ate: _____

_____

Snack _____

Who I ate with: _____

How I felt before/during/after I ate: _____

_____

Dinner: _____

Who I ate with: _____

How I felt before/during/after I ate: _____

_____

_____

Snack:_____

Who I ate with: _____

How I felt before/during/after I ate: _____

_____

What I did today that counts as exercise (in addition to my daily

activities) include how long: _____

_____

## DAY 51 Date_____ Weight_____

Oz of Lemon Water drank today _____

Breakfast: _____

Who I ate with: _____

How I felt before/during/after I ate: _____

_____

Snack:_____

Who I ate with: _____

How I felt before/during/after I ate: _____

_____

Lunch: _____

Who I ate with: _____

How I felt before/during/after I ate: _____

_____

Snack _____

Who I ate with: _____

How I felt before/during/after I ate: _____

_____

Dinner: _____

Who I ate with: _____

How I felt before/during/after I ate: _____

_____

_____

Snack:_____

Who I ate with: _____

How I felt before/during/after I ate: _____

_____

What I did today that counts as exercise (in addition to my daily
activities) include how long: _____

_____

## DAY 52 Date_____ Weight_____

Oz of Lemon Water drank today _____

Breakfast: _____

Who I ate with: _____

How I felt before/during/after I ate: _____

_____

Snack:_____

Who I ate with: _____

How I felt before/during/after I ate: _____

_____

Lunch: _____

Who I ate with: _____

How I felt before/during/after I ate: _____

_____

Snack _____

Who I ate with: _____

How I felt before/during/after I ate: _____

_____

Dinner: _____

Who I ate with: _____

How I felt before/during/after I ate: _____

_____

_____

Snack:_____

Who I ate with: _____

How I felt before/during/after I ate: _____

_____

What I did today that counts as exercise (in addition to my daily
activities) include how long: _____

_____

## DAY 53 Date_____ Weight_____

Oz of Lemon Water drank today _____

Breakfast: _____

Who I ate with: _____

How I felt before/during/after I ate: _____

_____

Snack:_____

Who I ate with: _____

How I felt before/during/after I ate: _____

_____

Lunch: _____

Who I ate with: _____

How I felt before/during/after I ate: _____

_____

Snack _____

Who I ate with: _____

How I felt before/during/after I ate: _____

_____

Dinner: _____

Who I ate with: _____

How I felt before/during/after I ate: _____

_____

_____

Snack:_____

Who I ate with: _____

How I felt before/during/after I ate: _____

_____

What I did today that counts as exercise (in addition to my daily

activities) include how long: _____

_____

**DAY  54  Date_____Weight_____**

Oz of  Lemon Water drank today _____

Breakfast: _____

Who I ate with: _____

How I felt before/during/after I ate: _____

_____

Snack:_____

Who I ate with: _____

How I felt before/during/after I ate: _____

_____

Lunch: _____

Who I ate with: _____

How I felt before/during/after I ate: _____

_____

Snack _____

Who I ate with: _____

How I felt before/during/after I ate: _____

_____

Dinner: _____

Who I ate with: _____

How I felt before/during/after I ate: _____

_____

_____

Snack:_____

Who I ate with: _____

How I felt before/during/after I ate: _____

_____

What I did today that counts as exercise (in addition to my daily
activities) include how long: _____

_____

## DAY 55 Date_____ Weight_____

Oz of Lemon Water drank today _____

Breakfast: _____

Who I ate with: _____

How I felt before/during/after I ate: _____

_____

Snack:_____

Who I ate with: _____

How I felt before/during/after I ate: _____

_____

Lunch: _____

Who I ate with: _____

How I felt before/during/after I ate: _____

_____

Snack _____

Who I ate with: _____

How I felt before/during/after I ate: _____

_____

Dinner: _____

Who I ate with: _____

How I felt before/during/after I ate: _____

_____

_____

Snack:_____

Who I ate with: _____

How I felt before/during/after I ate: _____

_____

What I did today that counts as exercise (in addition to my daily

activities) include how long: _____

_____

**DAY  56  Date_____ Weight_____**

Oz of  Lemon Water drank today _____

Breakfast: _____

Who I ate with: _____

How I felt before/during/after I ate: _____

_____

Snack:_____

Who I ate with: _____

How I felt before/during/after I ate: _____

_____

Lunch: _____

Who I ate with: _____

How I felt before/during/after I ate: _____

_____

Snack _____

Who I ate with: _____

How I felt before/during/after I ate: _____

_____

Dinner: _____

Who I ate with: _____

How I felt before/during/after I ate: _____

_____

_____

Snack:_____

Who I ate with: _____

How I felt before/during/after I ate: _____

_____

What I did today that counts as exercise (in addition to my daily

activities) include how long: _____

_____

**DAY 57   Date_____   Weight_____**

Oz of Lemon Water drank today _____

Breakfast: _____

Who I ate with: _____

How I felt before/during/after I ate: _____

_____

Snack:_____

Who I ate with: _____

How I felt before/during/after I ate: _____

_____

Lunch: _____

Who I ate with: _____

How I felt before/during/after I ate: _____

_____

Snack _____

Who I ate with: _____

How I felt before/during/after I ate: _____

_____

Dinner: _____

Who I ate with: _____

How I felt before/during/after I ate: _____

_____

_____

Snack:_____

Who I ate with: _____

How I felt before/during/after I ate: _____

_____

What I did today that counts as exercise (in addition to my daily

activities) include how long: _____

_____

## DAY 58    Date_____    Weight_____

Oz of Lemon Water drank today _____

Breakfast: _____

Who I ate with: _____

How I felt before/during/after I ate: _____

_____

Snack:_____

Who I ate with: _____

How I felt before/during/after I ate: _____

_____

Lunch: _____

Who I ate with: _____

How I felt before/during/after I ate: _____

_____

Snack _____

Who I ate with: _____

How I felt before/during/after I ate: _____

_____

Dinner: _____

Who I ate with: _____

How I felt before/during/after I ate: _____

_____

_____

Snack:_____

Who I ate with: _____

How I felt before/during/after I ate: _____

_____

What I did today that counts as exercise (in addition to my daily

activities) include how long: _____

_____

## DAY 59   Date _____ Weight _____

Oz of Lemon Water drank today _____

Breakfast: _____

Who I ate with: _____

How I felt before/during/after I ate: _____

_____

Snack:_____

Who I ate with: _____

How I felt before/during/after I ate: _____

_____

Lunch: _____

Who I ate with: _____

How I felt before/during/after I ate: _____

_____

Snack _____

Who I ate with: _____

How I felt before/during/after I ate: _____

_____

Dinner: _____

Who I ate with: _____

How I felt before/during/after I ate: _____

_____

_____

Snack:_____

Who I ate with: _____

How I felt before/during/after I ate: _____

_____

What I did today that counts as exercise (in addition to my daily

activities) include how long: _____

_____

## DAY 60 Date_____ Weight_____

Oz of Lemon Water drank today _____

Breakfast: _____

Who I ate with: _____

How I felt before/during/after I ate: _____

_____

Snack:_____

Who I ate with: _____

How I felt before/during/after I ate: _____

_____

Lunch: _____

Who I ate with: _____

How I felt before/during/after I ate: _____

_____

Snack _____

Who I ate with: _____

How I felt before/during/after I ate: _____

_____

Dinner: _____

Who I ate with: _____

How I felt before/during/after I ate: _____

_____

_____

Snack:_____

Who I ate with: _____

How I felt before/during/after I ate: _____

_____

What I did today that counts as exercise (in addition to my daily
activities) include how long: _____

_____

## DAY 61   Date_____ Weight_____

Oz of Lemon Water drank today _____

Breakfast: _____

Who I ate with: _____

How I felt before/during/after I ate: _____

_____

Snack:_____

Who I ate with: _____

How I felt before/during/after I ate: _____

_____

Lunch: _____

Who I ate with: _____

How I felt before/during/after I ate: _____

_____

Snack _____

Who I ate with: _____

How I felt before/during/after I ate: _____

_____

Dinner: _____

Who I ate with: _____

How I felt before/during/after I ate: _____

_____

_____

Snack:_____

Who I ate with: _____

How I felt before/during/after I ate: _____

_____

What I did today that counts as exercise (in addition to my daily
activities) include how long: _____

_____

## DAY 62   Date_____ Weight_____

Oz of Lemon Water drank today _____

Breakfast: _____

Who I ate with: _____

How I felt before/during/after I ate: _____

_____

Snack:_____

Who I ate with: _____

How I felt before/during/after I ate: _____

_____

Lunch: _____

Who I ate with: _____

How I felt before/during/after I ate: _____

_____

Snack _____

Who I ate with: _____

How I felt before/during/after I ate: _____

_____

Dinner: _____

Who I ate with: _____

How I felt before/during/after I ate: _____

_____

_____

Snack:_____

Who I ate with: _____

How I felt before/during/after I ate: _____

_____

What I did today that counts as exercise (in addition to my daily

activities) include how long: _____

_____

CONGRATULATIONS!

You've been Doin' It for 2 months!

Reward Yourself!!

If you haven't reached your Long Term Goal Order another workbook and just continue DOIN' IT!

If you HAVE reached your goal- Congratulations and enjoy the wonderful gift of health, and fitness that YOU just gave yourself!!

Keep this book as a keepsake of your road to success!

Read your inspirational thoughts often!

Don't forget all the things you've learned about yourself.

Keep your 'Tool Box' handy and watch out for those triggering situations and events.

Stay connected to your Support Team and any online or group supports that you've connected with.

Beware of the 'false friends' who would love nothing better than to bully you back into the mold where THEY were comfortable having you. Remember you've done this for yourself.!

## You deserve to be fit, healthy & thin!

If you catch yourself gathering any more excess baggage weather in the form of old tapes or fat JUST LET GO!

You may also enjoy 15-4-6 by Kit DeCanti which is no sweat routine which she developed and put on CD and DVD. Check out her website for more information

www.kitdeeproductions.com

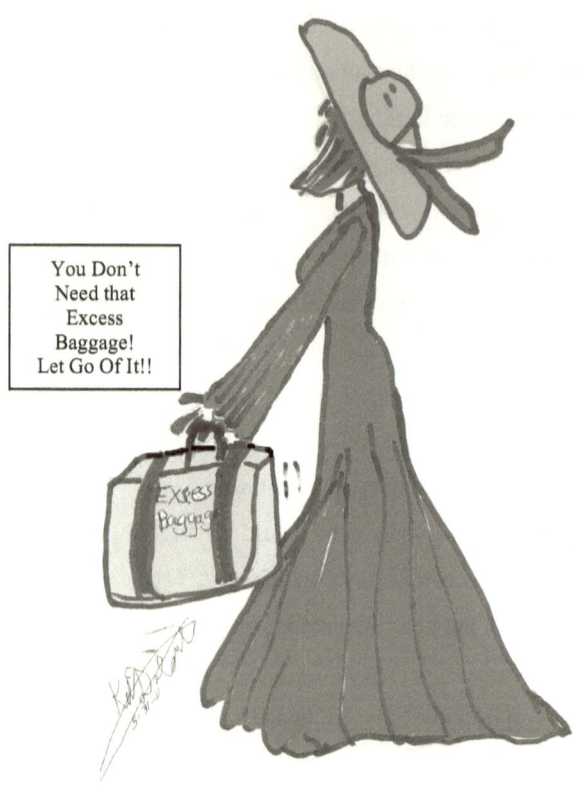

**You Deserve to be Healthy Fit & Thin**

**\*For a complete photo record of**

**author's journey to Healthy, Fit & Thin**

**go to www.kitdeeproductions.com**